Dear reader,

"***How to Live Disease-Free with Superfoods***" *aims to provide you with in-depth knowledge about superfoods that have medicinal effects and can help prevent and control diseases naturally.*

Eat healthy, live happy!

Master of Pharmacy,

Registered Pharmacist

and Research Scientist

How to Live Disease-Free with SUPERFOODS

A Complete Superfoods Guide for Healthy Living

LA FONCEUR

Eb
emerald books

Eb
emerald books

This book has been published with all efforts taken to make the material error-free. The information on this book is not intended or implied to be a substitute for diagnosis, prognosis, treatment, prescription, and/or dietary advice from a licensed health professional. Author doesn't assume and hereby disclaim any liability to any party for any loss, damage, or disruption caused by errors or omissions, whether such errors or omissions result from negligence, accident, or any other cause.

While every effort has been made to avoid any mistake or omission, this publication is being sold on the condition and understanding that neither the author nor the publishers or printers would be liable in any manner to any person by reason of any mistake or omission in this publication or for any action taken or omitted to be taken or advice rendered or accepted on the basis of this work.

CONTENTS

INTRODUCTION

Nowadays, chronic diseases such as diabetes, high blood pressure, and arthritis have become quite common. One in every family has one of these diseases. People have started considering these diseases as part of life, which is not good. The lifestyle we are leading today - high intake of processed foods, frequent eating out, smoking, and alcohol, there is a 70% chance that you will have either high blood sugar levels or high blood pressure or both by your 50s.

A disease state in the body means your immune system is constantly busy fighting the disease, soon your immune system loses its effectiveness and becomes weak. If another disease strikes, your immune system is unable to fight, this can have life-threatening consequences. It is very important to start as early as in your 20s to take care of your health. Make your body strong enough to fight any disease naturally.

More diseases mean more medicines. Being from a pharmacy background, I can assure you that dependence on medicines is not good. Medicines prescribed in disease have side effects. To reduce side effects, you are often prescribed with another set of medicines that treat the side effects of your primary medications, but they also have side effects, for which again some other medications are required, so basically, this cycle continues. But there is a solution! You can include foods in your diet that have the same effect as your medications. By regular intake of these foods, you can heal your body and increase your immunity to fight disease naturally.

The objective should be to prevent disease, and preparation starts in your 20s. What you eat in your 20s affects your 50s. To prevent a disease, you must have a thorough knowledge of the disease, such as why it happens? How does it affect your body? What exactly does happen in your body in the event of a disease? What are other health problems that can be caused by a particular disease?

In ***How to Live Disease-Free with Superfoods***, all these topics will be discussed in detail. You will learn about foods that boost your immunity, superfoods that can protect you from diseases, foods that reduce inflammation in your body, and food combinations that you should eat for maximum health benefits. Get ready for a healthy tomorrow!

1

ROLE OF FOOD THERAPY IN PREVENTING AND CONTROLLING DISEASE

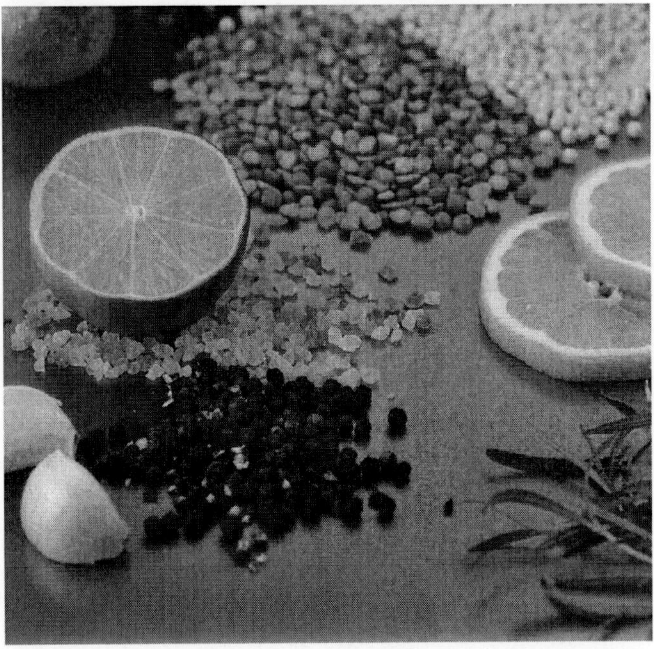

Role of food therapy in preventing and controlling disease

If you have your blood sugar levels checked for the first time, and your report says that your blood sugar is high, your doctor will not first prescribe you the medicines. Instead, your doctor will give you a three-month time so that you can control your sugar with diet and lifestyle modifications. If the blood sugar is still not controlled, then only you will be prescribed with medicines to control high sugar levels.

You know why? Because medicines treat disease, but they can cause strong side effects. The stronger the drug, the stronger will be its side effects. It doesn't mean you should stop taking medicines without informing your doctor. Never stop your medication without consulting your doctor because some medicines have withdrawal effects, which can even worsen your disease condition if you stop taking them suddenly.

So, what is the solution? The solution lies in good management. You can prevent or manage the disease only when you have comprehensive knowledge about that disease. Everything is on your hand, and you are the commander of your life and your disease condition. With the correct nutrition and healthy lifestyle, you require fewer medicines, shorter therapy duration, and minimum side effects.

When it comes to disease management, there are lots of misconceptions associated with it. Let's first clear these misconceptions:

#1 Misconception

I am young, and I don't have any disease, I have plenty of time to live without worrying. I will worry about diseases when I will hit my 50. Till then, my motto is *You Only Live Once*.

Actually, you only die once but live every day, so make your every day disease-free. The age of 20 to 40 is your key to make your 50+ years healthy and happy. The way you treat your body between these years, its effect is seen in your old age. These are your sowing years, eat as many healthy foods as you can during these years, and reap the benefits in your 50+ years. Strictly avoid smoking, alcohol, and other drugs that deteriorate your health internally. The harm never visible during your 20s and 30s, but it has life-threatening consequences soon after you hit your 50s or nowadays even in your 40s. Eat junk foods but only to satisfy your taste bud, definitely not to fill your tummy.

#2 Misconception

I am a very health-conscious person, and I believe nature has all the solutions. Although I have been diagnosed with a disease, but I believe I don't need medication. I can heal myself naturally with healthy food and a good lifestyle.

If you have been diagnosed with a disease means the harm has unknowingly already been done. Keep in mind medicines are not the enemy, just they are not a natural food. Sole dependence on medicines is not good; at the same time, completely abandoning medicines when your body needs them is also not right. No doubt, healthy foods, and healthy lifestyle choices can heal you much faster, but you definitely need medication to treat a disease. With healthy foods, you can heal yourself faster, and your body recovers more quickly, so you need a shorter course of therapy that simply means lesser side effects.

#3 Misconception

Last time when I had these symptoms, my doctor prescribed these medicines. Now again, I feel the same problem, I should take the same medicines as the doctor had prescribed me last time.

Avoid self-medication. In a condition of reoccurrence of any disease, medicines may be the same, but with different doses. Don't be a doctor yourself. Self-medication may result in an overdose, which can lead to toxicity and other life-threatening consequences. Seek advice from your doctor every time you are not feeling well and ask him/her directly if it is safe to take the same medication again when the symptoms occur. Always ask your doctor about what should be the diet in managing your disease? Ask your pharmacist if there is any food that you should avoid while taking the prescribed medicine.

#4 Misconception

I was on medication, and my condition has improved. Although my doctor had prescribed me a 3-month course of medicines, I was feeling fine, so after two months, I stopped taking the medicines.

This is never advised. Maybe with your healthy diet and lifestyle, you have recovered faster than others, but you should never leave your medication course in between without consulting your doctor. Even if your symptoms are relieved with initial medications, you need the full course to treat the disease completely. Otherwise, it will reoccur, and as it has not been treated in the initial stage, it will reoccur with more severeness. Abruptly discontinuing some medicines produce withdrawal effects in the body and worsen the disease condition. Instead of quitting your medicines, you should inform your doctor about your improvement. Your doctor will gradually reduce the dose of the same medication and complete the course sooner than before, or he will advise you to complete the full course depending upon your disease type and your condition.

#5 Misconception

I am taking medicine for my illness, and medicine is doing its job. It will cure me, I don't have to worry too much about nutrition and all.

Food and lifestyle play a huge role in managing any disease. If your diet is not healthy and your lifestyle is also not good, then your condition may worsen despite regular medication. Foods that boost immunity prepare your body to fight the disease and heal your body. A healthy lifestyle removes the burden from your body; hence your body can completely focus on treating the disease.

#6 Misconception

Some diseases like diabetes, high blood pressure, arthritis, etc. come naturally with age. You cannot escape from these diseases. Every other person I know has one of these diseases, so this is pretty normal at my age.

It may be common but indeed not normal. This is the biggest myth that some diseases naturally come with age. With age, our body becomes a little weaker, but most of these diseases are the result of our poor diet and poor lifestyle. It's time to stop letting these diseases become part of your life and build your body with healthy foods and a healthy lifestyle in such a way that these diseases never even touch you, and if you already have these diseases, then they can be controlled.

DISEASE MANAGEMENT

What is a disease?

A disease is a condition of disturbances in the normal structure or function of your body. When something goes wrong with the normal function of your body, your body gives signals in the form of signs and symptoms that something is going wrong inside the body. This is where your responsibility begins. With proper medication, healthy foods, and healthy lifestyle, you can prevent and treat disease.

Disease is mainly managed with medications and foods and lifestyle modifications. Let's understand the role of each.

ROLE OF MEDICATIONS

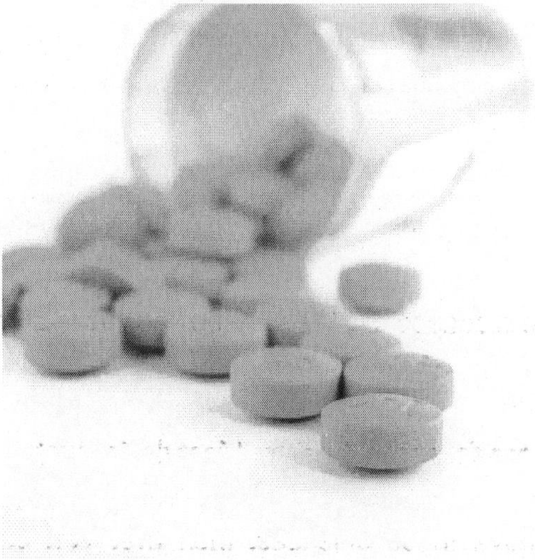

Prescribed medications play a vital role in the treatment. Generally, medicines work in three ways:

1. To reduce symptoms like pain, nausea, and fever.

2. To treat the disease.

3. To reduce or treat the side effects arising due to the use of medicines in curing the disease. Such as antacids are usually prescribed with high dose medications as these medications can cause acidity in the body.

It is important to take the medicines at the same time every day. Medicines take their time (onset time) to show their effect on the body. Taking medicines at the same time every day ensures that its active ingredient will be available in the body uniformly throughout the treatment.

ROLE OF LIFESTYLE CHOICES

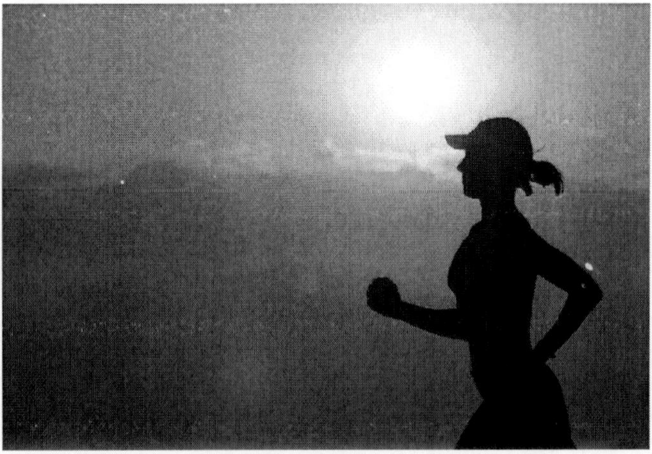

Poor lifestyle choices give a burden to your body. In simple terms, these are the inducer of many diseases. Unhealthy lifestyle choices weaken your body, lower your immunity, and make you susceptible to many diseases.

Example of unhealthy lifestyle choices:

- Stress
- Smoking
- Alcohol
- Unhygienic habits
- Inadequate sleep

When it comes to poor lifestyle choices, you may have found plenty of discussions about smoking, alcohol, and inadequate sleep, but we often take other poor lifestyle choices such as stress and unhygienic habits lightly.

Stress is a key contributor to many diseases. When you are under stress, your body releases the stress hormone cortisol, which causes your heart to pump faster and raises your blood pressure. After the stressful time has passed, your body releases lower amounts of cortisol. Your heart and blood pressure return to normal. But if you are under constant stress, the consistently high levels of cortisol in your body can cause many health problems. Take out at least 2 hours for yourself every day, do nothing during this time, just relax. Just two stress-free hours in a day gives your body enough time to normalize all its functions and systems.

Unhygienic habits such as not washing your hands before eating and after using the washroom, and touching an open wound allow germs to enter the body. As a result, your immune system keeps busy fighting these germs and with time immune system weakens. When your immune system becomes weak, it can't protect you from major and serious diseases. So, don't stress out your immune system. Already there is so much pollution in the environment with which your immune system fights daily, so do not give it more burden. Maintain good hygiene and keep your immune system healthy. Whenever you come from outside, first wash your hands with soap water. This habit will protect you from many diseases. Also, 5-Second rule is a big myth. Even a brief exposure of the floor can contaminate your food with E. coli, salmonella, and other bacteria in under five seconds.

What should be your focus points to prevent disease?

If you keep your immune system and digestive system healthy, you greatly lower your risk of diseases.

Avoid Immune weakening lifestyle choices

- Stress
- Smoking

- Drinking Alcohol
- Consuming narcotics such as Cannabis

Adapt the immune-boosting lifestyle choices

- 7-8 hours of sleep
- Washing your hands frequently
- Expose yourself to early morning sunlight
- Yoga
- Taking a walk after lunch and dinner

Avoid immune weakening foods

- Trans fats
- Processed foods
- Canned foods
- Refined carbohydrates
- Foods high in sugar

Add immune-boosting foods in your diet

- Foods rich in vitamin C
- Foods high in zinc
- Foods that have anti-inflammatory effects

ROLE OF FOODS

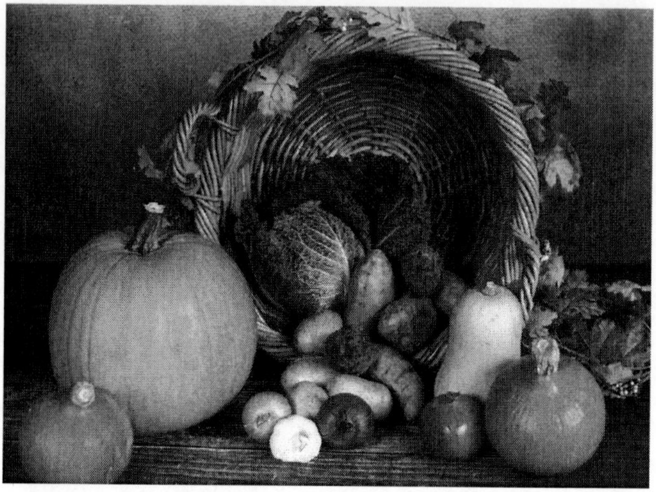

Foods play a massive role in every stage of disease management. These roles include:

1. To prevent the disease.
2. To shorten the therapy period.
3. To control the disease.
4. To prevent the reoccurrence of the disease.

Body is nature's product, and your body loves natural things like food. Plant-based healthy foods can prevent various diseases and autoimmune disorders and help build your body strong enough to fight off any disease. Plant-based healthy foods heal your body, reduce your dependency on medicines, and add disease-free years to your life.

Why food therapy is the best therapy?

Medicines work on the disturbance that has been arisen in your body dues to disease, while foods work on the root cause and strengthen your body to fight with the disease naturally. Moreover, foods have no side effects. A simple rule is to include vegetables and fruits of every color in your diet; it will protect you from countless diseases.

We are so concerned about avoiding unhealthy foods that it has become quite stressful now. The more you try to run away from them, the more you crave. If you do not eat unhealthy foods, but your diet lacks essential nutrients, then there is no health benefit of avoiding unhealthy foods. To stay healthy, incorporating healthy foods into your diet is more important than just avoiding unhealthy foods. It is time to focus on what you should eat, not what you should not eat. Do not modify your diet for weight loss; instead, balance your diet for a healthy and disease-free life.

2

10 SUPERFOODS YOU MUST EAT EVERY DAY TO LIVE DISEASE-FREE

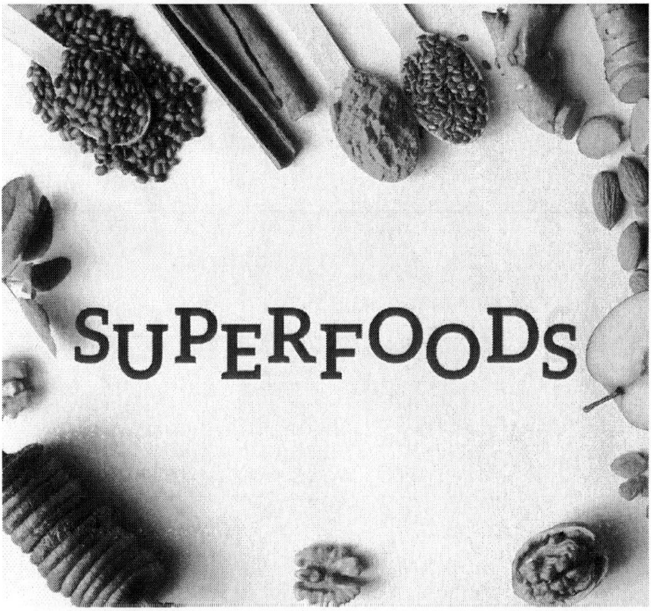

10 superfoods you must eat every day to live disease-free

Foods can protect you from many diseases and can improve your disease condition. Superfoods are foods that are highly dense in nutrients. A food is considered as a superfood when it not only can protect or treat a single disease, but its regular consumption can protect you against many diseases at a time. Eating just superfoods and avoiding other foods doesn't guaranty you a disease-free life. But eating superfoods every day definitely reduces the risk of developing the disease manifold. This is because superfoods contain active chemical compounds that are antioxidant and anti-inflammatory, and inhibit oxidative stress by killing free radicals and reduce inflammation in the body. Oxidative stress and inflammation are the leading causes of cancer, arthritis, diabetes, and many such chronic diseases. You can prevent these diseases by eating superfoods every day. Do not look at superfoods as medicines that you only need until your condition improves. See them as lifelong friends; They are here to do good for you, so you must keep their company throughout life. I am listing top superfoods that you must include in your everyday diet. But to stay disease-free, you should also avoid eating processed foods, canned foods, fried items, salt, and other well-known health deteriorators. Here are superfoods that have medicinal properties and can reduce your dependency on medicines. Let's meet our lifelong food friends:

TURMERIC

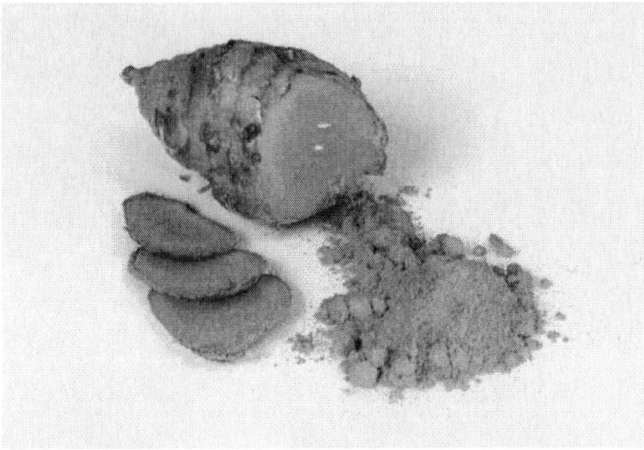

Turmeric deserves to be at the top of the superfoods list. Turmeric has scientifically proven health benefits. The credit goes to curcumin, the active compound of turmeric. Curcumin gives the bright yellow color to turmeric and has many medicinal properties. It is a potent anti-inflammatory, antioxidant, antibacterial, antiviral, and antifungal agent. These properties play an important role in keeping your body strong enough from inside to prevent most of the disease.

Inflammation is good for the body as it helps heal an injury or fights infection, but our today's food and lifestyle cause inflammation in the body at a dangerous level. Chronic inflammation is one of the reasons for almost every disease, including arthritis, heart disease, Alzheimer's disease, depression, cancer, and other degenerative conditions. Curcumin has potent anti-inflammatory property which protects you from many diseases. Lower levels of Brain-Derived Neurotrophic Factor (BDNF) is associated with Alzheimer's and depression. Turmeric boosts the levels of BDNF and very effective in preventing and treating depression and Alzheimer's disease.

Turmeric helps prevent and control a variety of cancer types, including prostate, breast, colorectal, and pancreatic cancers. It helps stop the growth of tumor cells.

Due to its antibacterial and antiviral property, curcumin might help fight off infection and a variety of viruses, including herpes and viral flu. So, next time when you get a viral fever, add one tablespoon of turmeric powder in milk, boil for two minutes, and drink it before bed. It will heal you faster.

Turmeric protects cells from the damage caused by free radicals. Unhealthy foods like foods high in saturated fats, sugar as well as poor lifestyle choices such as drinking alcohol contribute to free radicals, which is associated with tissue damage. Free radicals can cause damage to cells of DNA, proteins, and cell membranes, by pairing with their electrons through the oxidation process. These are responsible for aging and other health complications. Turmeric has a high content of polyphenols, flavonoids, tannins, and ascorbic acid; these all are the natural antioxidants and help protect cells from the damage caused by free radicals.

How to consume turmeric?

Eat fresh turmeric in the winter season. Grate it and add in your morning tea. In other seasons, use turmeric powder in cooking and have hot turmeric milk at night before bed. Turmeric is warm in nature, so don't overeat it in summer, you may get mouth ulcer.

Who should avoid turmeric?

No one. It can consume by anyone. Eat black pepper with turmeric; it increases curcumin absorption in the body. However, if you are taking blood-thinning medicines like warfarin, you should limit your turmeric consumption because turmeric purifies the blood and thins the blood.

How much turmeric should I eat in a day?

You should aim to get 500mg-1000mg of curcumin in a day, which is equivalent to one tablespoon of freshly ground turmeric or one tablespoon of turmeric powder. Avoid supplements rather than go for fresh or powdered turmeric.

FENUGREEK LEAVES AND SEEDS

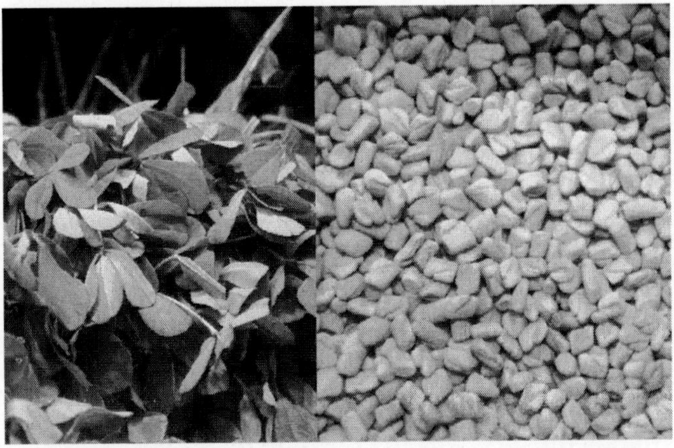

Fenugreek leaves and seeds have a wide range of nutrients that provide numerous health benefits. They are packed with iron, vitamins, biotin, choline, flavonoids, and fibers. The high antioxidant flavonoid content in fenugreek seeds can reduce pain and inflammation and improve arthritis conditions. Fenugreek leaves and seeds are high in soluble fiber, which helps lower blood sugar and decreases cholesterol levels. The fiber in fenugreek slows down the digestion and absorption of carbohydrates and is very effective in controlling diabetes. High blood cholesterol levels increase your risk of heart diseases. The soluble fiber in fenugreek gets attached to cholesterol particles and takes them out from the body, thus decreasing the cholesterol levels in the body and reduces blood pressure. This reduces the risk of developing heart complications and improves heart health.

Also, fenugreek seeds are effective in the treatment of hair loss, male impotence, and other types of sexual dysfunction.

How much fenugreek should I consume in a day?

One teaspoon of fenugreek seeds in a day for six months to see the result. Aim to eat fresh fenugreek leaves every day or every alternate day in the winter season.

What is the best way to consume fenugreek?

Soak one teaspoon of fenugreek seeds in a glass of water overnight. Next morning, chew the fenugreek seeds and swallow them with a full glass of water (in which seeds were soaked). Make fresh fenugreek leaves salad or sauté them in mustard oil, add garlic to enhance the taste.

Who should avoid fenugreek?

If you are on medication of diabetes or hypertension, don't start taking fenugreek in high amount without consulting your doctor and pharmacist. Fenugreek may perform similar functions as your diabetes and BP medications. So taking both may lower blood glucose and blood pressure below the safe range. Because of that, the dose of your medicines might need to be changed.

FLAX SEEDS

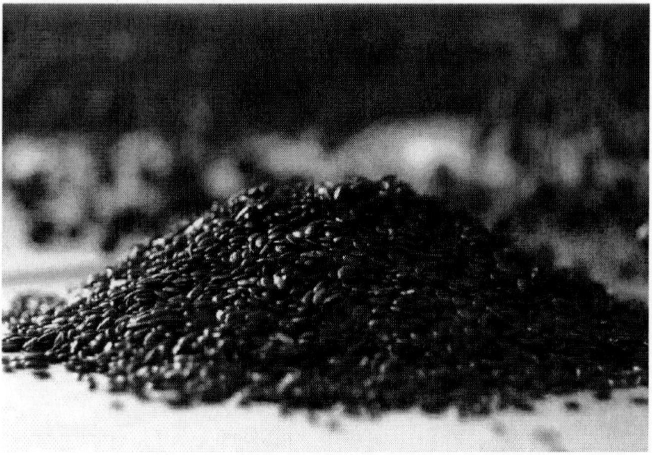

Flax seeds are probably the healthiest among all the seeds. They have got the reputation of superfood because they are packed with cancer-fighting polyphenols lignans, alpha-linolenic acid (ALA), and fibers. Flax seeds contain approximately 100 times more lignans than any other plant foods, which helps in protecting against breast cancer, colon cancer, and prostate cancer. They are one of the best sources of an omega-3 fatty called acid alpha-linolenic acid (ALA). Due to their high omega-3 content, they help reduce the risk of heart disease, stroke, and diabetes through their anti-inflammatory action. Omega-3 fatty acid alpha-linolenic acids, along with lignans, block the release of pro-inflammatory agents and reduce inflammation in the body. The anti-cancer property of flax seeds is due to their lignans content; they suppress the growth, size, and spread of cancer cells by blocking enzymes that are involved in hormone metabolism.

How much flax seeds should I eat in a day?

One tablespoon (10g-15g) of flax seeds in a day.

What is the best way to eat flax seeds?

Dry roast and grind them. Add the ground flax seeds in chapati and tortilla dough.

Who should avoid flax seeds?

There are no side effects reported till date, so it is safe to eat flax seeds for all. Always remember moderation is the key. Consuming too much flax seeds with too little water can worsen constipation and may lead to an intestinal blockage, so take flax seeds with plenty of water to prevent this from happening.

SWEET POTATOES

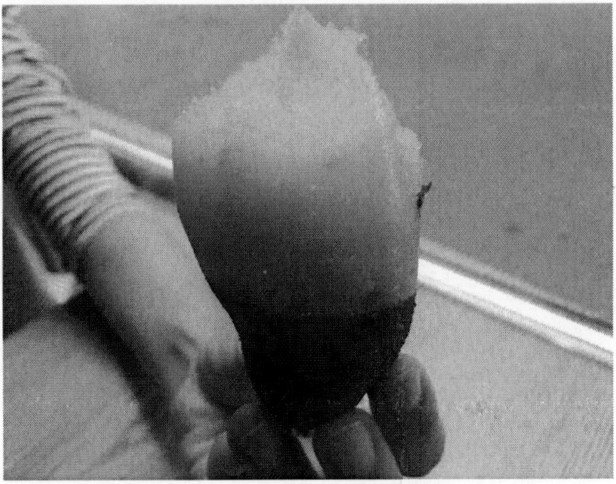

Sweet potatoes are one of the best sources of beta carotene that converts into vitamin A in the body and promote eye health as well as boost immunity. Beta carotene functions as a potent antioxidant that reduces cell damage and helps prevent the free radical damage that is associated with cancer. The higher fiber content of sweet potatoes prevents constipation and promotes a well-functioning digestive tract. The presence of anthocyanin pigments in sweet potatoes, particularly in purple-fleshed sweet potatoes, helps in preventing and reducing chronic inflammation in the body.

Sweet potatoes are rich in both magnesium and potassium, both of which are essential in lowering blood pressure and reduce the risk of cardiovascular diseases.

Higher fiber and magnesium content of sweet potatoes may decrease diabetes risk. Moreover, sweet potatoes help to regulate the blood sugar levels, especially in people with diabetes; its high insoluble fibers content promotes insulin sensitivity. Unlike other starchy foods, sweet potatoes have a low glycemic index. They release sugar into the bloodstream slowly and steady, which aids in controlling the blood sugar levels of individuals.

How many sweet potatoes should I eat in a day?

One medium sweet potato in a day is enough to meet your daily recommended vitamin A intake.

What is the best way to cook sweet potatoes?

To get the most nutrition from your sweet potatoes, don't peel them, simply wash, and scrub well before cooking. They can be boiled, steamed, and baked. Steamed or boiled sweet potatoes have more healthy benefits than baked sweet potatoes because baking releases the sugar inside the sweet potato, which may increase blood glucose levels.

Who should avoid eating sweet potatoes?

People who have existing kidney stones or are at high risk of developing them or those who are on dialysis should avoid sweet potatoes. It is because sweet potatoes are high in potassium, and when you have kidney disease, your kidneys cannot remove extra potassium, and too much potassium can stay in your blood.

COW'S MILK

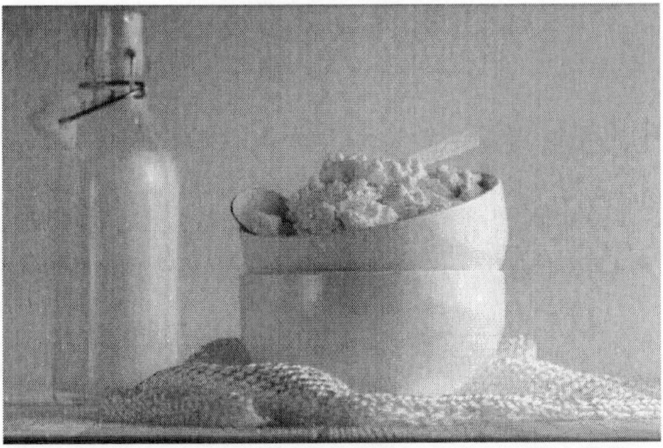

The reason why you should drink milk every day is because cow's milk is a complete food means it contains every nutrient that you need in a day for a healthy body. Cow's milk is packed with protein, calcium, potassium, vitamin A, B vitamins, and phosphorous. When you feel hungry, have a glass of cow's milk, it's enough to give you energy for the next 2 -3 hours.

Let's see why milk is so good for your health:

Amino acids are compounds that combine to make proteins. Your body needs nine essential amino acids through food to maintain normal functioning. Not all protein sources are considered as a high-quality complete protein because not all protein-rich foods contain all nine essential amino acids. Milk is a rich source of protein, mainly casein (80%) and whey (20%). Both are considered as complete protein because both contain all nine essential amino acids that are required for your body to maintain good health.

Milk is an excellent source of calcium, which is necessary to build healthy bones and teeth and to maintain bone mass. The presence of vitamin D in milk increases the absorption of calcium in the body. Calcium with vitamin D can protect you from osteoporosis.

Magnesium and potassium in milk support proper kidney and heart function and can help you prevent hypertension and heart diseases.

Milk is a complete package; you can get all essential nutrients in a single, convenient source. If you are thinking of switching to vegan, keep in mind that it is hard to have all milk's nutrients in a single vegan food source. Most of the vegan sources are fortified means extra nutrients are manually added to them, and these nutrients are not naturally present in them, so basically, these are not natural sources. Also, when you switch to vegan, you need supplements to reach daily vitamins and minerals need of the body, which is an effective way but again, not the natural way. Anything which is not natural is not advised to be dependent on for a long time.

Milk products that you should add in your diet:

Cow's milk (best for health), low-fat yogurt, buttermilk, cottage cheese, and cow's milk's ghee.

Milk products that you should avoid:

Heavy cream, processed cheese, and whole-fat dairy products.

How much milk and milk products should I consume in a day?

250 ml cow's milk + 2-3 milk products (yogurt, cottage cheese).

Who should avoid milk?

If you are lactose intolerant, you should avoid milk. Another alternative is lactose-free cow's milk, which contains all the nutrients of milk, but it's free from lactose. Lactose-free cow's milk is made by adding the enzyme lactase to cow's milk, which breaks down the lactose into glucose and makes it lactose-free and can easily be digested by lactose-intolerant people.

Limit your dairy consumption in the wet season. Consuming too much dairy can aggravate gastric problems, cause nausea, diarrhea, and stomach pains, even though if you are not lactose intolerant. So, moderation is the key.

If you have a cough, limit your milk and milk product consumption. Avoid taking milk at night. Milk doesn't increase the production of phlegm, but it can make your existing phlegm thicker and may irritate your throat and aggravate a cough.

RAW GARLIC

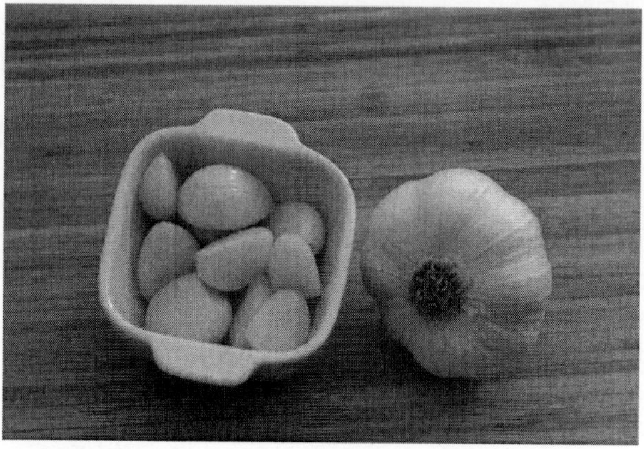

Garlic is an adaptogen which means it stabilizes and maintains a steady internal environment in the body, in response to environmental changes. It ensures the optimal functioning of the body, including the regulation of body temperature, blood sugar, blood pressure, pH balance, and functioning of the immune system. This is the reason why initially garlic had used for medicinal purposes only. Most of the potent medicinal properties of garlic are due to the allicin, a sulfur compound that gives pungent smell to the garlic. The thing with allicin is that it only releases when you crush or cut the garlic. Allicin is very unstable, which means you need to use it immediately after you cut garlic. The allicin in raw crushed garlic is destroyed by heat. So, for health benefits, eat fresh raw garlic.

Also, garlic protects against bowel and stomach cancers. It is scientifically proven that the sulfur components of garlic alter the biological behavior of tumors, tumor microenvironments, and precancerous cells. Garlic decreases cancer risk, particularly cancers of the gastrointestinal tract.

Garlic is known to contain natural antioxidants that can eliminate low-density lipoprotein (LDL) cholesterol from the body and help protect against heart disease by thinning the blood and improve blood circulation. Garlic reduces both systolic and diastolic blood pressure by increasing the nitric oxide production in the body, which helps smooth muscles to relax and widen the blood vessels.

The antibacterial and antifungal properties of garlic help fight infections and boost the function of the immune system. So basically, this vegetable (yes, it's vegetable, not an herb or spice) can actually protect you from many diseases. It's time to add RAW garlic in your diet!

How should I take garlic?

Eat one clove of freshly crushed raw garlic every morning on an empty stomach. Don't eat more than one clove of fresh raw garlic at a time. Don't keep garlic in the mouth for too long; it may cause burn. Eat plenty of garlic (raw and cooked) in winter, add them in soup or spring roll. Limit garlic consumption in the summer season, too much of garlic in summer, may result in acne and ulcer due to its heat-producing nature.

When should I avoid garlic?

If you have ulcers, colitis, acid reflux, or heartburn problem, limit your garlic consumption.

How much garlic is enough for health benefits?

One clove of raw garlic (crushed) on an empty stomach every day is enough. If you experience heat, ulcer or acid reflux, then instead of daily, eat it twice or thrice a week.

SPROUTS

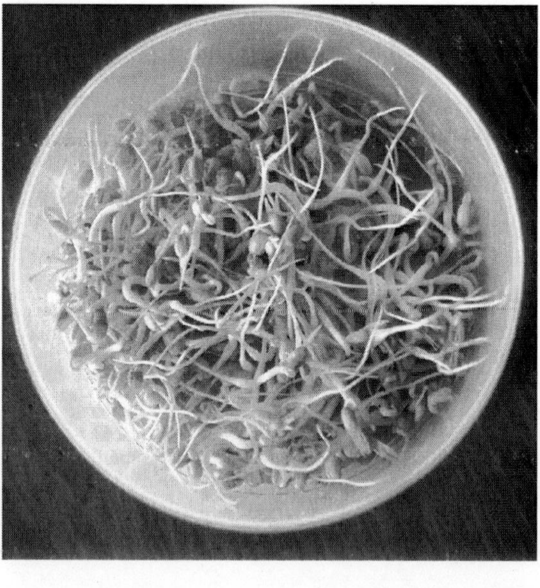

Sprouts are affordable, safe, and easily grown nutrient-dense superfood. Sprouting can increase nutrition up to 100 times than raw legumes and vegetables.

For those who have difficulty digesting certain foods, sprouting is a better option for them. The reason is sprouting increases the proteolytic enzymes content of the food that break down starches into simpler carbohydrates, proteins into amino acids, and fats into fatty acids. So, your digestive system need not break them, which makes these nutrients more bioavailable and easily digestible.

Why is sprouting beneficial for you? Because sprouting increases the nutrition value of legumes and vegetables, it removes enzyme inhibitors and unlocked healthy compounds. The increased bioavailability of high levels of vitamins, minerals, amino acids, essential fatty acids, and antioxidants increases the alkalinity of your body. Raising pH (to an alkaline state) increases the ability of your immune system to prevent disease.

Grow sprouts at your home to reduce your exposure to pesticides, food additives, and other chemicals. There are so many different sprouts varieties you can try, including mung bean, black chickpeas, lentils, wheat sprouts, alfalfa, radish seeds, and broccoli.

How many sprouts should I eat in a day?

Eat a bowl of different varieties of sprouts in a day. You don't need to eat the same sprouts every day, keep them rotating, eat every sprout on alternate or every three days, but try to have a bowl of sprouts every day.

What is the best way to eat sprouts?

Eating them raw will keep all the nutrients locked. To make them tangy, add finely chopped cucumbers, onions, tomatoes, fresh-squeezed lemon juice, black salt, and black pepper.

Who should avoid eating sprouts?

In case you are going for store-bought sprouts (which I would not recommend at all), don't eat them raw. Cook them thoroughly until steaming hot throughout to reduce the risk of food poisoning from Salmonella, Listeria, or E. coli. Store-bought sprouts can be contaminated anywhere along the journey from farm to table. People with weakened immune systems should not eat any variety of raw or lightly-cooked sprouts; it may result in food poisoning.

SPINACH

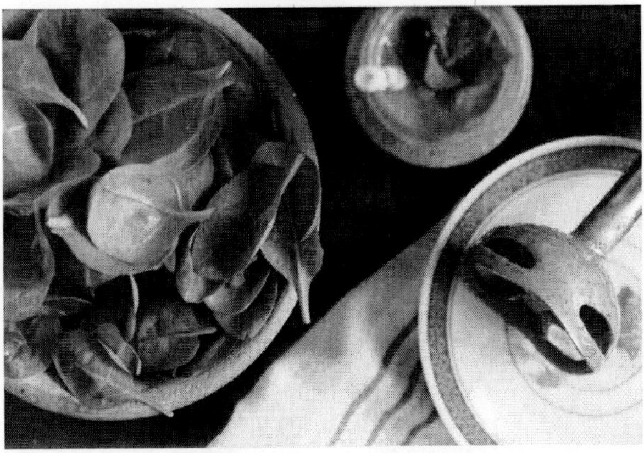

Spinach is called a superfood because of its anti-inflammatory and antioxidant properties. It is packed with iron, vitamin k, protein, calcium, magnesium, and potassium that protect your body from a wide range of diseases. Spinach is a significant source of vitamin K, which is an important factor in wound healing and bone health. Spinach is rich in carotenoids that are beneficial antioxidants that boost your immune system. It contains three different types of carotenoids: beta carotenoid, lutein, and zeaxanthin.

Beta carotenoid converts into vitamin A in the body and has a vital role in maintaining healthy vision, healthy immune system, and healthy reproduction system. Lutein and zeaxanthin function as a light filter, protecting your eye tissues from UV rays of sunlight.

The high levels of potassium in spinach, along with folate, relaxes the blood vessels and lower your blood pressure. Spinach also helps the body make nitric oxide, a natural vasodilator which further lowers blood pressure.

Often people who have type 2 diabetes have low levels of magnesium. Spinach is very low in calories and has a low glycemic index. Additionally, it is rich in magnesium, which helps to lower blood sugar and can even protect you from type 2 diabetes.

What is the best way of eating spinach?

The more you cook spinach, the more it will lose its nutrients. Either sauté the spinach or blanch the spinach, but don't blanch for more than 1 minute. Add lemon juice while blanching, it will increase the absorption of nutrients in your body, and you will get the full health benefit.

Who should not eat spinach?

Limit your spinach consumption if you have kidneys stone or if you are at a high risk of developing kidney stones because spinach is high in both calcium and oxalates that can cause kidney stones.

If you are taking blood-thinning medication, do let your doctor and pharmacist know about your spinach consumption. Spinach is high in vitamin K that promotes blood clotting and can decrease the effectiveness of your blood-thinning medication such as warfarin.

DRY FRUITS

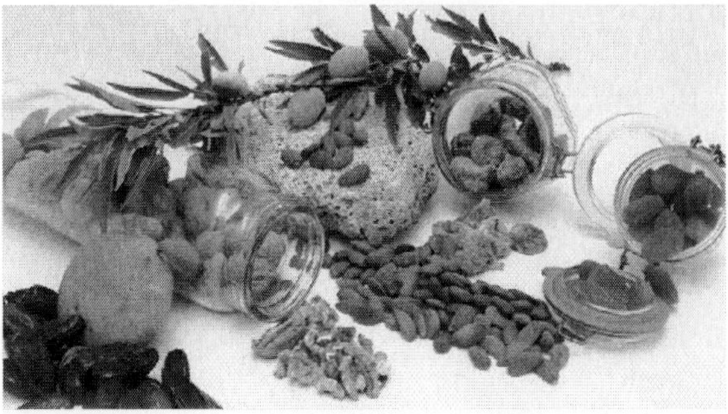

You must have heard this 1000 times that you should eat nuts every day! But do you follow it? If not, then it's time to start eating nuts every day! Eating dry fruits every day helps promote overall well-being and ensures a healthy, disease-free long life. Nuts contain heart-friendly monounsaturated and polyunsaturated fats, and antioxidants like flavonoids and vitamin E. Research suggests that high consumption of nuts, including peanuts, is associated with two to three times reduced risk of breast cancer.

Dry fruits are high in fiber and magnesium, which help to stabilize blood sugar and insulin levels. Dry fruits lower the risk of developing type 2 diabetes.

Dates are loaded with iron and potassium and yet contain little sodium, which helps maintain normal blood pressure and keeps the risk of a stroke in check.

Dried figs are a good source of calcium. Figs keep bodily systems like the endocrine, immune, respiratory, digestive, and reproductive system in check.

Almonds are an excellent source of vitamin E, protein, and monounsaturated fats. They promote weight loss by reducing hunger and keeping you full for a longer period. The healthy fats and antioxidants of almond lower blood pressure and cholesterol levels and also lower the blood sugar levels.

Walnut kernels don't just look like a brain, but they actually contain brain-boosting polyphenolic compounds like omega-3 fatty acids. Polyphenols are considered critical brain food and prevent cognitive disorders.

Cashew nuts are rich in zinc, which boost immunity and prevent male pattern baldness and prostate enlargement by blocking the creation of Dihydrotestosterone (DHT).

How many dry fruits should I eat in a day?

Eat a handful of different dry fruits every day, including almond, walnut, cashew nuts, pistachio, dates, raisins, and figs. Frequency matters, so it is important to eat them every day even if the quantity is less than a handful.

What is the best way to eat dry fruits?

Nuts contain phytic acid that reduces the nutrition value of nuts by lowering absorption, so the best way to remove phytic acid is soaking. Soak a handful of dry fruits in water overnight and eat them the next morning.

Who should avoid eating dry fruits?

You should eat plenty of dry fruits in winter but limit your dry fruits consumption in the summer season. Nuts produce heat in the body, while it is beneficial in winter to keep you warm; in summer, it can give you acne, ulcer, and acidity.

BASIL LEAVES

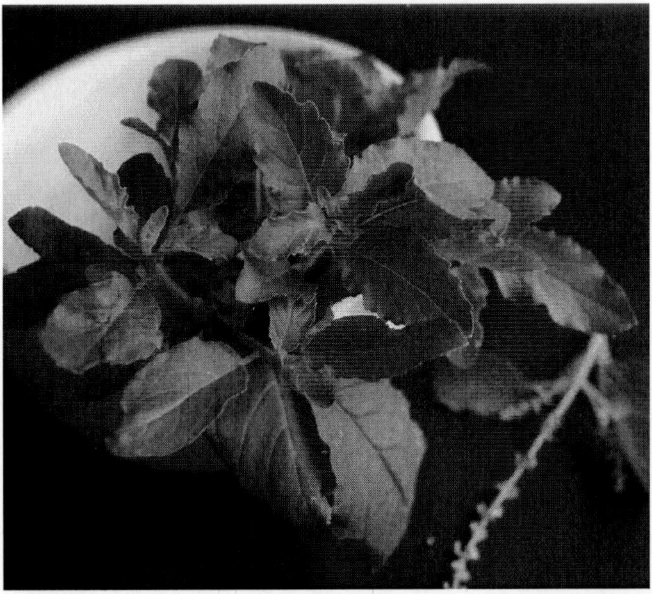

Holy basil or tulsi is a superfood because it is an immunomodulator and adaptogen. It lowers blood sugar levels, cholesterol, and triglycerides.

Stress increases your risk of developing or worsens conditions like hypertension, diabetes, heart disease, Alzheimer's disease, depression, obesity, and gastrointestinal problems. Adaptogen with anti-inflammatory properties of basil helps you to reduce stress, anxiety, depression, and very effective in preventing and treating cognitive disorders, including amnesia and dementia. The neuroprotective, anti-stress, and anti-inflammatory activities of basil enhance memory and improve brain function. For this reason, basil considers as a natural memory tonic.

Regular consumption of basil leaves can prevent viral infections. Research confirms that holy basil has an immunomodulatory effect; it increases the percentage of T-helper cells as well as NK-cells (Natural killer cells), which are the components of the adaptive immune system and innate immune system, respectively. These cells help eliminate pathogens by preventing their growth and help fight viral infections.

Research shows basil leaves are as effective in lowering blood glucose as antidiabetic drugs. Basil leaves have hypoglycemic properties, which lower blood sugar levels and improve insulin sensitivity. If you have prediabetes or type 2 diabetes, the essential oil of basil helps cut down cholesterol and triglyceride levels, which is a persistent risk factor for type 2 diabetes.

How much basil should I consume in a day?

Start your day by chewing two to three fresh basil leaves.

What is the best way to eat basil leaves?

Add 2-3 fresh basil leaves in your morning green tea. You don't need much expertise in growing basil at your home.

Who should avoid eating basil leaves?

Limit your basil consumption if you are taking medications like acetaminophen or paracetamol (pain reliever). If you are consuming plenty of basil leaves and taking paracetamol, they both work together and tend to affect the functioning of your liver.

CONCLUSION

Now that you know the foods that can naturally protect you from diseases, should you just opt for their dietary supplement? Not at all. Supplements are never recommended in place of natural foods. This is because the supplements contain ingredients that have strong biological effects in the body. Their dose may interfere with medications you may already be taking, which can sometimes have harmful consequences. Taking too much of some supplements can have life-threatening consequences. You should include various natural foods in your diet, not human-made foods, so supplements are a big no in replacing superfoods.

3

10 POWER FOODS TO BOOST YOUR IMMUNITY

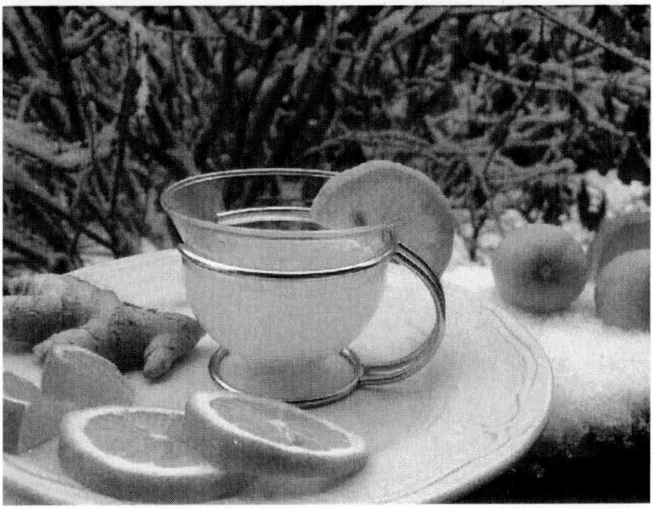

10 power foods to boost your immunity

Keeping your immune system healthy, directly means protecting yourself from many diseases. In winter, cold and flu are quite common but have you ever thought why few people get flu while others not. The reason is their immunity. Some people have a naturally strong immune system, while others have weak. No matter whether your immunity is naturally strong or weak, you can definitely boost your immunity with some power foods. This will not only make your winter flu-free, but it will also protect you from many diseases.

When it comes to immunity, the four major nutrients that need to be taken into consideration are as follow:

Vitamin C is the most crucial nutrient for boosting your immunity. Vitamin C supports various cellular functions of the immune system, thus contributes to immune defense.

Vitamin A promotes as well as regulates the immune system. Therefore, it enhances the immune function and provides an enhanced defense against multiple infectious diseases.

Vitamin E is a potent antioxidant and can modulate immune functions. Studies suggest vitamin E improves the decreased immunity in aged people.

Omega-3 fatty acids are anti-inflammatory means they prevent inflammation or swelling in the body.

Zinc is an essential mineral that is crucial for the normal development and function of cells mediating immunity.

These five nutrients are crucial for maintaining and boosting immunity. A deficiency in any of these nutrients may weaken your immune system. Eating foods rich in zinc, omega-3, vitamin A, C, and E, help you build a stronger immune system. Let's see which power foods contain an abundance of these crucial nutrients.

Below are the 10 power foods to boost your immunity, so, start adding them in your diet for a disease-free, healthier life:

1. Citrus fruits

If you think of immunity, the first name that comes in your mind is vitamin C! and why not? Vitamin C is actually the best nutrient when it comes to immunity. It protects against immune system deficiencies, skin wrinkling, cardiovascular disease, eye disease, etc. Vitamin C increases the production of white blood cells, which are an essential part of the immune system. These are the key to fight infections by killing bacteria and viruses that invade the body. Citrus fruits such as lemon, tangerine, orange, and grapefruit are high in Vitamin C.

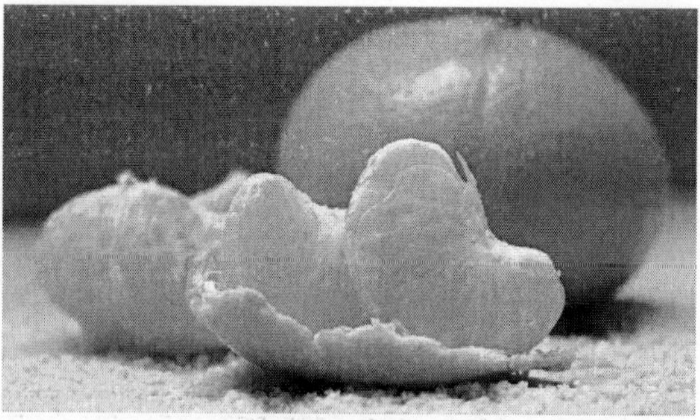

Citrus fruits are a natural antioxidant that boosts the immune system. These have antiviral and antibacterial properties that prevent infections, bacterial growth, and relieves nausea.

Squeeze one medium lemon in one glass of warm water (250 ml) and drink it every morning. You need vitamin C daily for continued health, so make a habit of taking lemon water instead of plain water every morning.

2. Turmeric

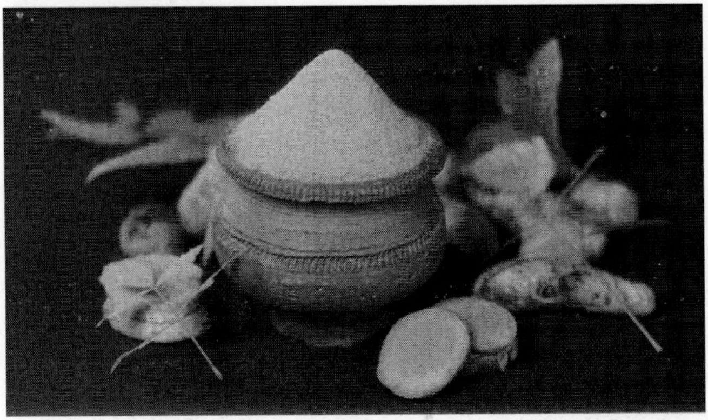

This bright yellow spice is a natural immunomodulator that boosts your immunity. Curcumin, the active compound of turmeric has many scientifically-proven health benefits. Curcumin is a potent antioxidant and has anti-inflammatory effects. Turmeric not only boost your immunity but also very effective in treating both rheumatoid arthritis and osteoarthritis. Add one tablespoon of turmeric powder in hot milk (250 ml) and drink it every night just before bed and see the magic yourself.

3. Garlic

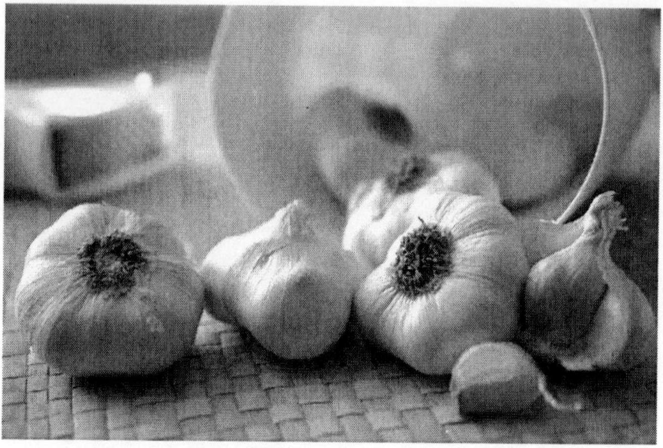

Garlic is an adaptogen, which means it helps the body to adapt varied environmental and psychological stresses and supports all the major systems, such as the nervous system, immune system, and hormonal system. It regulates blood sugar; if they are too high, it will lower it and vice-versa.

Garlic contains active compound allicin that improves the immune cells' ability to fight off the flu and reduces the risk of infection. Garlic also has anti-inflammatory, antibacterial, and antiviral properties that help in inhibiting the growth of some bacteria and fight against viral infections.

Taking one clove of crushed garlic on an empty stomach every day not only boosts your immunity but also normalizes all major systems in your body. If your body is already acidic or warm in nature, limit the consumption to 3 times a week.

4. Ginger

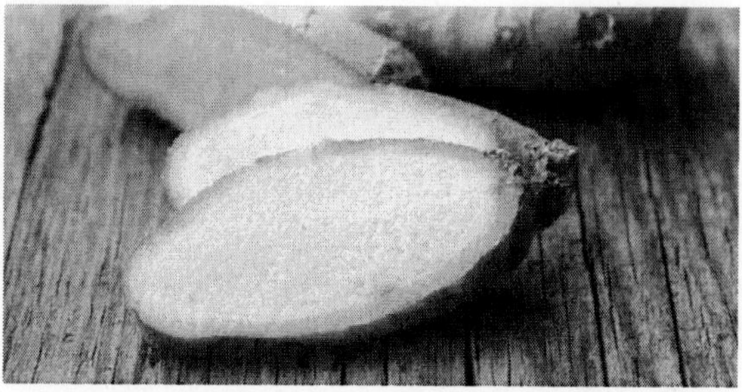

The bioactive substance gingerol in the ginger root has anti-inflammatory and anti-fungal properties. It helps in lowering the risk of infections and relieving a sore throat. It also helps fight viruses such as rhinoviruses, human respiratory syncytial virus (HRSV), which cause colds, and many respiratory infections. Ginger is a strong antioxidant, it naturally boosts your immunity. Drinking ginger tea every morning in the winter season keeps you warm and saves you from cold and flu.

5. Flax seeds

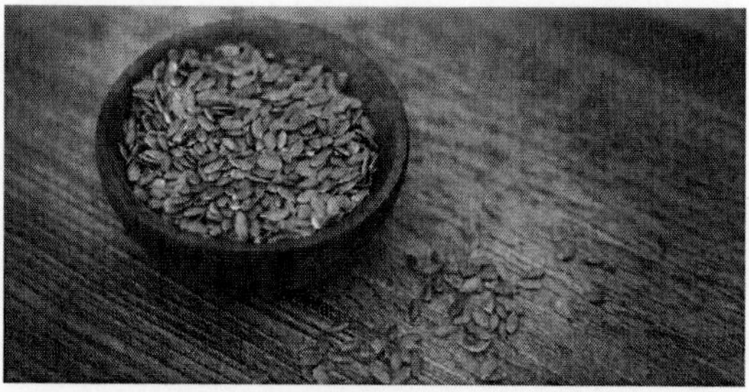

Flax seeds are rich in Omega-3 fats that help protect your body against bacteria and viruses, improving your immunity. Flax seeds contain the highest concentrations of dietary lignans that help protect against cancer by blocking the growth and spread of tumor cells. These are also a great source of iron that ensures your immune system gets required oxygen to fight infection. The omega-3 fatty acids of flax seeds fight inflammation in the body and prevent inflammatory diseases such as rheumatoid arthritis, psoriasis, and lupus.

6. Red and green bell peppers

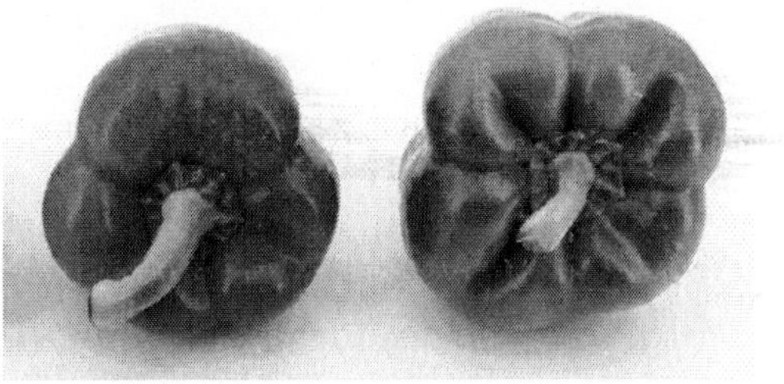

If you think orange or lemon is the richest source of vitamin C, then here is the surprise, bell peppers contain twice as much vitamin C as any citrus fruit. They are also a rich source of beta carotene, which converts into vitamin A in your body. The high content of both vitamin C and vitamin A in bell peppers enhance your immune function and provide enhanced defense against multiple infectious diseases. Vitamin A is an anti-inflammation vitamin that helps in treating and preventing arthritis and contact dermatitis. Eat cooked bell peppers because cooking increases vitamin C content in bell peppers.

7. Cashews

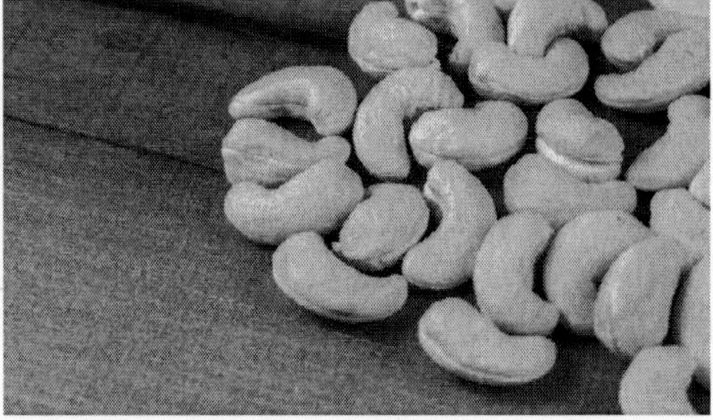

Cashews are a great source of zinc and copper. Zinc plays an important role in the production of immune cells and antioxidant enzymes that help fight disease and infection. Cashews have antioxidant effects that help your body fight off oxidative damage. Cashews speed up the healing of wounds as they are rich in vitamin K. Vitamin E of cashews help decrease inflammation in your body. Pregnant women must eat cashews as they help with the growth and development of the baby.

8. Papaya

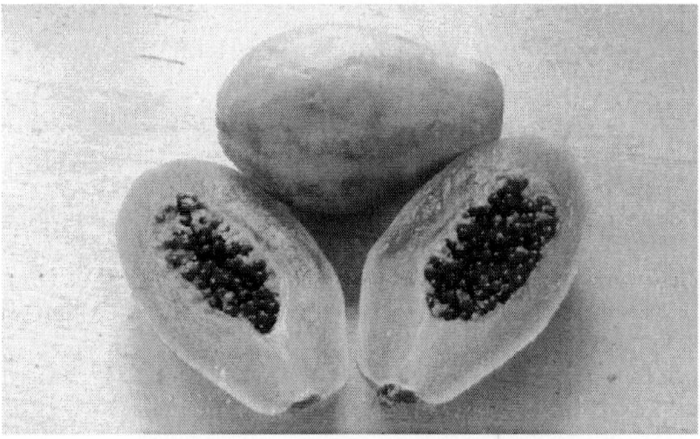

Papaya has antioxidant and immunostimulant effects that reduce oxidative stress and improve immune functions. Papayas also contain potent antioxidants known as carotenoids – particularly lycopene. Carotenoids are converted into vitamin A in the body and help regulate the immune system. Papaya is also a great source of vitamin B, C, and K and known as an excellent immunity booster. It slows down the aging process and helps your skin look more youthful and supple. One medium-sized papaya can fulfill your daily requirement of vitamin A.

9. Yogurt

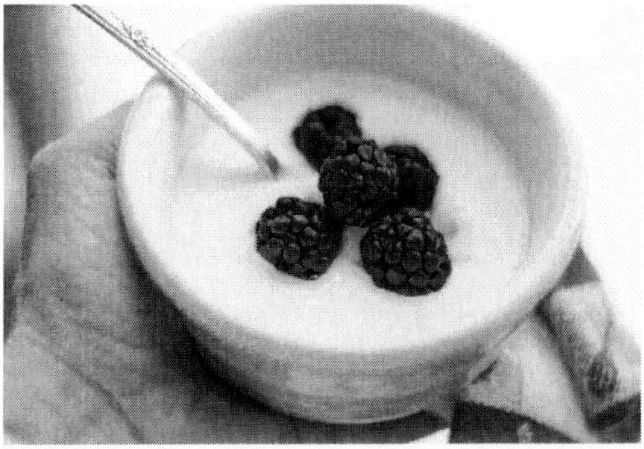

It is said that the healthier your gut is, the better will be your immunity. Yogurt is the best probiotic. Yogurt contains lactobacillus, a probiotic, or good bacteria that help keep your gut healthy, also gives your immune system a boost. Yogurt is also high with vitamins and protein. Due to the immunostimulatory effects of yogurt, it helps fight against diseases such as infection, GI disorders, cancer, and asthma. It is actually very beneficial for older people. Go for plain yogurt, not the flavored ones, and eat it with your lunch.

10. Green tea

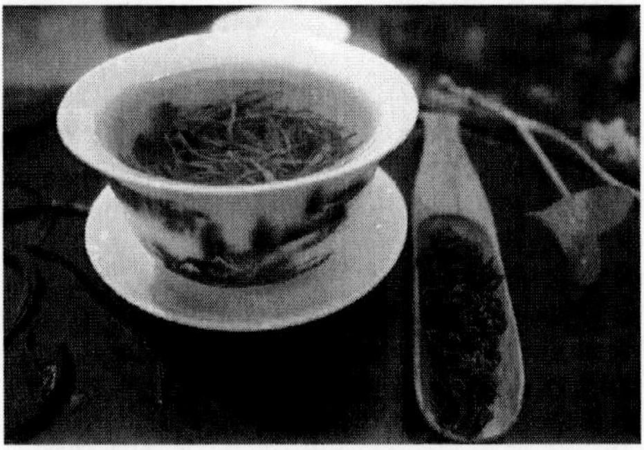

The list is incomplete without the mention of green tea. The higher concentration of polyphenols and flavonoids, the two powerful antioxidants, make green tea a gem for boosting your immunity. These antioxidants kill the free radicals in the body and increase your longevity.

Free radicals are the by-products of the process where cells use oxygen to generate energy in the body. At low or moderate levels, free radicals are harmless, but at high concentrations, they cause oxidative stress, a deleterious process that can damage all cell structures. Oxidative stress plays a crucial role in the development of arthritis, autoimmune disorders, cancer, aging, cardiovascular and neurodegenerative diseases.

The powerful antioxidants in green tea kill these free radicals and help in fighting illnesses, like common cold, arthritis, aging, and cancer. Start drinking green tea if you have not started yet!

CONCLUSION

These foods definitely boost your immunity, but to keep your immune system healthy, it is also important to have a healthy lifestyle that includes getting sufficient sleep, doing yoga, taking a morning walk, and managing your stress. Definitely, there are dietary supplements available in the market to boost your immunity, but their effects are limited. One good thing about going natural is, it comes with all benefits with no side effects. Most of the immune booster foods also enhance your skin and hair health, so it's a win-win situation.

4

10 NUTRIENT COMBINATIONS YOU SHOULD EAT FOR MAXIMUM HEALTH BENEFITS

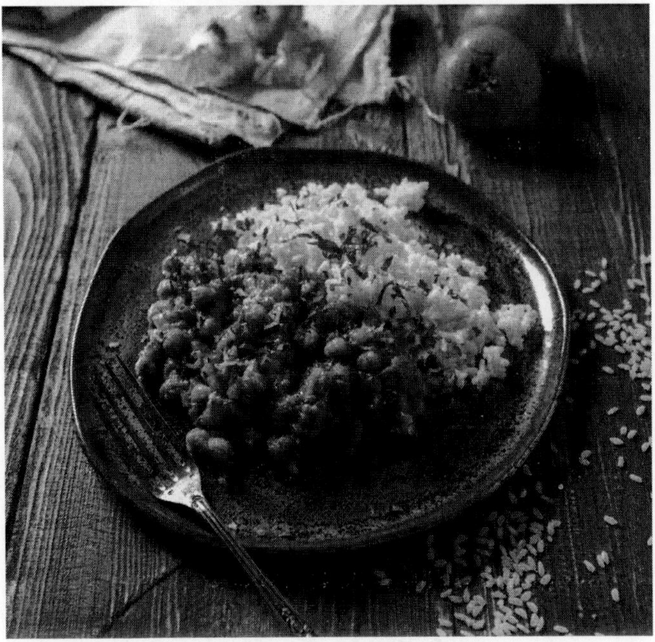

10 nutrient combinations you should eat for maximum health benefits

Nutrients need to adequately absorbed into your body to provide health benefits. Some nutrients are eliminated faster from your body without being absorbed, and you don't get their health benefits. Various factors affect the absorption of nutrients. Foods require a favorable environment inside your body and the presence of certain vitamins and minerals to get absorbed. If foods don't get absorbed in your body, you don't get the health benefits. Fortunately, you can enhance the absorption of food by pairing it with other food that can provide an environment required for their absorption and prevent their metabolism, making the nutrient more available in the blood to get absorbed. Eating these foods together ensures that you get maximum health benefits.

Below are 10 nutrient combinations that you should eat for maximum health benefits.

1. Vitamin C + Iron

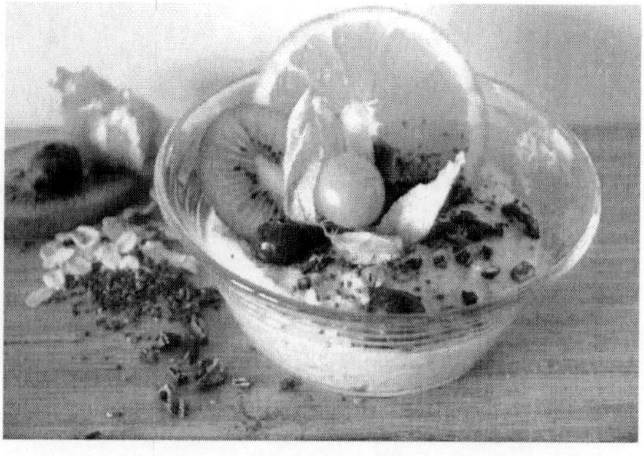

Iron is an essential nutrient required for blood production. Hemoglobin of red blood cells comprises about 70 percent of iron. Hemoglobin transfers oxygen through your blood from the lungs to the tissues. Deficiency in iron may cause iron-deficiency anemia that can lead to heart problems. You may become deficient in iron if you are eating too little iron-rich foods, or the iron is not getting absorbed properly in the body. When you eat vitamin C with iron, it increases the stability and solubility of iron by binding with them. Once iron becomes more soluble, it allows the body to more readily absorb the iron through the mucus membranes of the intestine.

Food combinations that you should eat for better iron absorption:

1. Lemon juice + Spinach

    Add lemon juice when blanching the spinach, it will retain the dark green color of spinach as well as increase the iron absorption.

2. Lemon juice + Sprouts

3. Tomatoes + Lentils

4. Orange + Oatmeal

5. Tomatoes + Beetroot

2. Vitamin D + Calcium

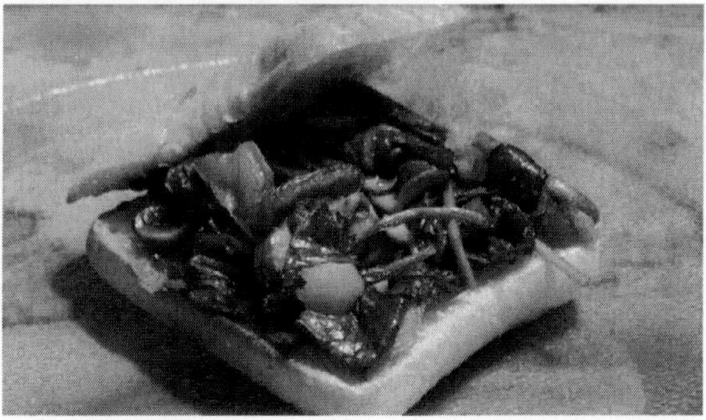

Calcium and vitamin D both are very important for your bone health. Not only your bones but your heart, muscles, and nerves also need calcium to function properly. You must have noticed that the prescribed calcium tablets always come in a combination of vitamin D. There is a solid reason behind it. Vitamin D is the fat-soluble nutrient that increases the absorption of calcium in the intestine. Calcium, along with vitamin D, not only can protect you against osteoporosis and bone disease. This combination can even protect against diabetes, high blood pressure, and cancer.

Food combinations that you should eat for better calcium absorption:

1. Expose your skin to sunlight for 10 to 15 mins in the morning after that drink a glass of milk.

2. Mushrooms + Soybeans

3. Yogurt + Nuts

4. Mushrooms + Dark leafy greens

5. Sour cream + Broccoli

3. Turmeric + Black pepper

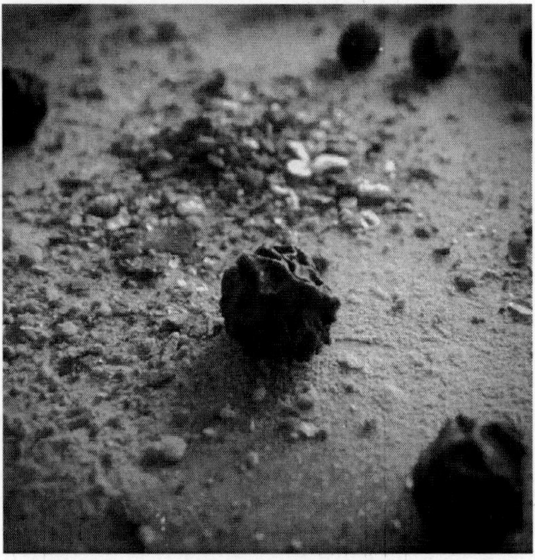

Turmeric has health benefits due to its active compound curcumin. The problem with curcumin is its poor absorption in the body. Additionally, curcumin is rapidly metabolized in the body that leads to its rapid elimination from the body. As a result, you could be missing out on its health benefits. By combining turmeric and black pepper, you can increase curcumin bioavailability. Black pepper has active ingredient piperine that protects curcumin from the digestive enzymes. It slows down the breakdown of curcumin. As a result, curcumin remains in the bloodstream for a longer period. It, therefore, boosts the absorption of curcumin by multiple times, making it more readily available to be used by the body.

4. Zinc + Vitamin A

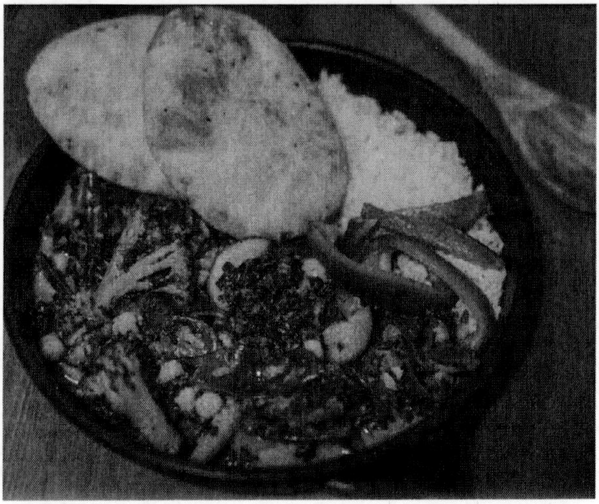

Vitamin A is not only crucial for protecting against night blindness, but it also promotes healthy growth and development and has a very critical role in enhancing immune function. Absorption of vitamin A is hugely affected by zinc availability in the body. Zinc plays a vital role in the absorption, transporting, and utilization of vitamin A in the body. When your body is deficient in zinc, it affects the movability of vitamin A from the liver to body tissues. Zinc also regulates the conversion of retinol (vitamin A) to retinal that requires the action of a zinc-dependent enzyme. So, if you eat vitamin A-rich foods together with zinc-rich foods, you will get the maximum health benefits of vitamin A.

Food combinations that you should eat for better vitamin A absorption:

1. Cashew nuts + Carrot cake
2. Legumes + Spinach
3. Dry fruits + Mango milkshake
4. Swiss cheese + Sweet potato
5. Oats + Papaya

5. Green tea + Lemon

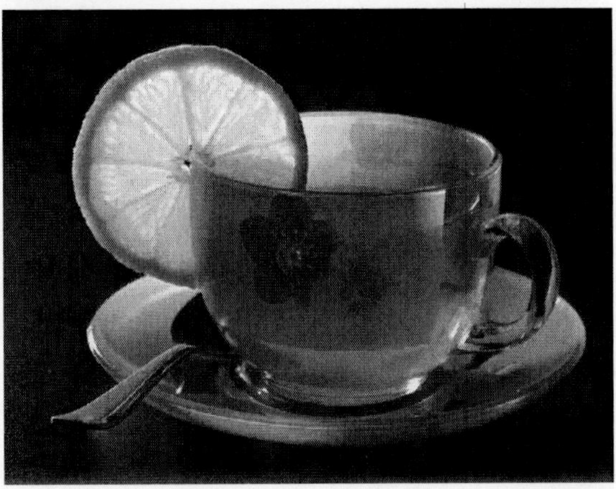

Green tea is loaded with catechins which are the polyphenols that have potent antioxidative, anti-inflammatory, and antibacterial activity. Catechins improve blood pressure, blood sugar levels, prevent cell damage and very effective in preventing cancer.

The catechins of green tea are relatively unstable in the intestine. Vitamin C rich foods such as citrus fruits increase the amount of catechins available for the body to absorb. Vitamin C interacts with catechins to prevent their degradation in the intestines. As a result, more catechins are available to absorbed in the body. So, make sure to add lemon juice in your green tea because when you add lemon in your green tea, it increases catechins absorption by more than five times.

6. Phytic acid + Water

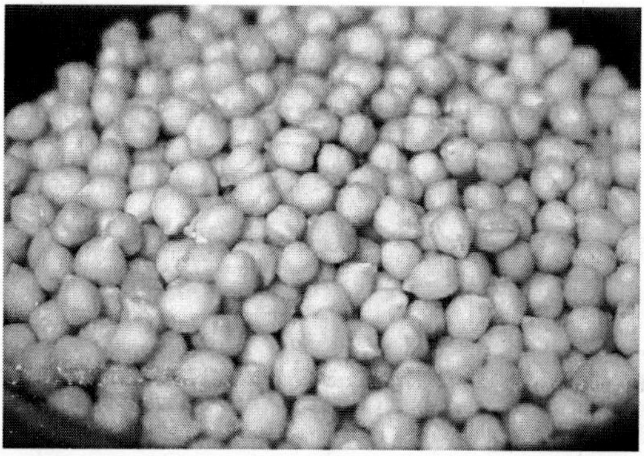

Plant-based foods such as whole grains, legumes, and nuts contain phytic acid that binds with minerals such as iron, zinc, calcium, and manganese and prevents their absorption in the body. When phytic acid binds with these minerals, it forms phytates, and our bodies do not have any enzymes that can break down phytates to release these minerals. So, you don't get the full health benefits of these minerals. Fortunately, the simple solution to this problem is soaking! Soaking in water allows the phytic acids to leach onto the water. You should soak phytic acid-containing foods in water overnight (or for at least 3-4 hours). It will increase the bioavailability of the minerals and decrease gastrointestinal distress.

Foods that you should soak for better absorption:

1. Nuts (Almond, peanuts, walnuts, and others)

2. Legumes (kidney beans, chickpeas, and peas)

3. Rice

4. Wheat bran

5. Sesame

7. Tomato + Olive oil

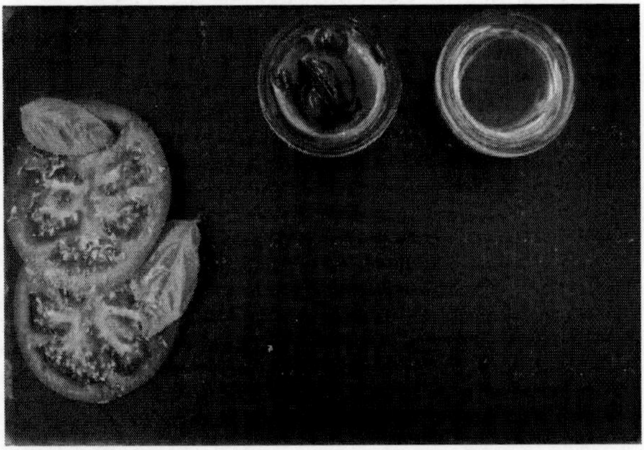

Lycopene is the main carotenoid in tomatoes. The antioxidant lycopene of tomatoes is responsible for reducing the risk of heart disease and certain types of cancer. Lycopene is a fat-soluble compound, which means it is better absorbed in the presence of healthy fat. Eating tomatoes cooked in olive oil greatly increase the absorption of lycopene and protect your cells against free radicals, which play a role in aging, heart disease, cancer, and other diseases.

8. Folate + Vitamin B12

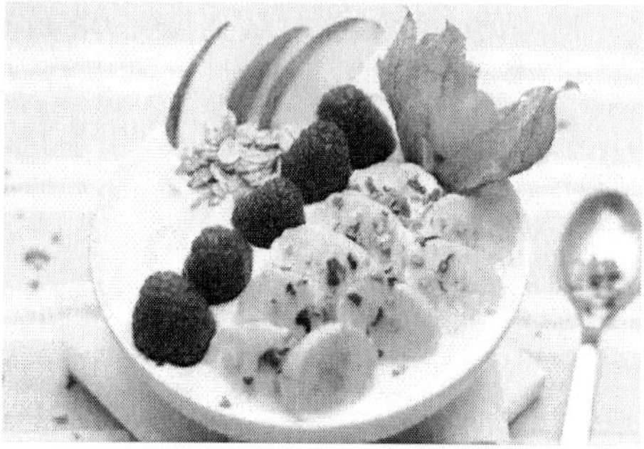

Folate (Folic acid or vitamin B9), when taken alone, can mask the symptoms of vitamin B12 deficiency. The problem is that without symptoms, you will not know that you are deficient in vitamin B12. This can delay the diagnosis, and there could be a risk of developing nerve damage. Because of this reason, these vitamins are often taken together. Moreover, folate works closely with vitamin B12 to make red blood cells and to help iron function properly in the body. Folate and vitamin B12 together (along with vitamin B6) help lower homocysteine levels. Study shows high levels of homocysteine (an amino acid) are associated with the development of coronary artery disease, leading to heart attacks and strokes. If you eat folate and vitamin B12 rich foods together, you will never get deficient in folate or vitamin B12, and you will never get depressed because these two vitamins, when eaten together, enhance the immune function and mood.

Folate and vitamin B12 food combinations that you should eat for maximum health benefits:

1. Yogurt + Banana
2. Shiitake mushrooms + Dark leafy greens
3. Milk + Nuts
4. Yogurt + cooked Okra (Ladyfinger)
5. Whey + Lentils

Whey is the by-product of cottage cheese-making. It is the liquid remaining after milk has been curdled and strained. Cook lentils in whey instead of plain water.

9. Rice + Beans (complete protein)

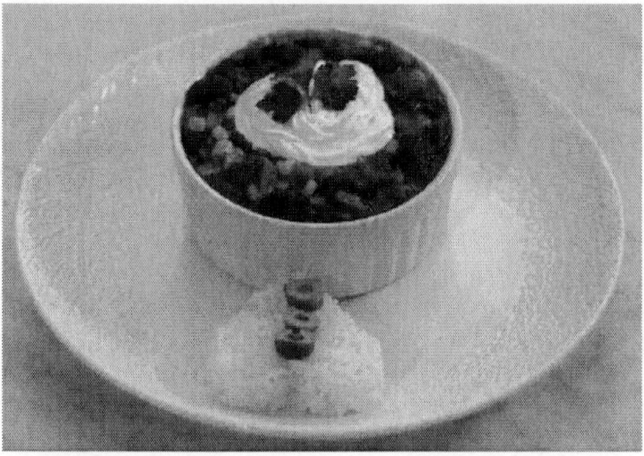

The human body needs nine amino acids, which are essential means you need to get them through food. A complete protein means a food source of protein that contains an adequate amount of each of the nine essential amino acids. Not all protein sources are a complete protein, especially vegetarian protein sources. That doesn't mean being a vegetarian, you will miss out on amino acids. When you eat correct food combinations, you can get all the essential amino acids. The best example is rice and beans. Together, rice and beans form a complete protein because when eaten together, they provide all nine essential amino acids necessary in the human diet.

Beans are rich in lysine but missing an amino acid known as methionine. Rice has high levels of methionine but doesn't have enough amino acid lysine. When rice and beans (such as kidney beans and chickpeas) are consumed together, each provides the amino acid that the other lacks, making it a high-quality protein. Here are some more high protein food combinations.

Food combinations that you should eat to get complete protein:

1. Kidney beans + Rice
2. Green peas + Lentils
3. Corn + Mixed beans
4. Red lentils + Brown rice
5. Cabbage + Wheat

10. Vitamins A, D, E and K + Healthy fats

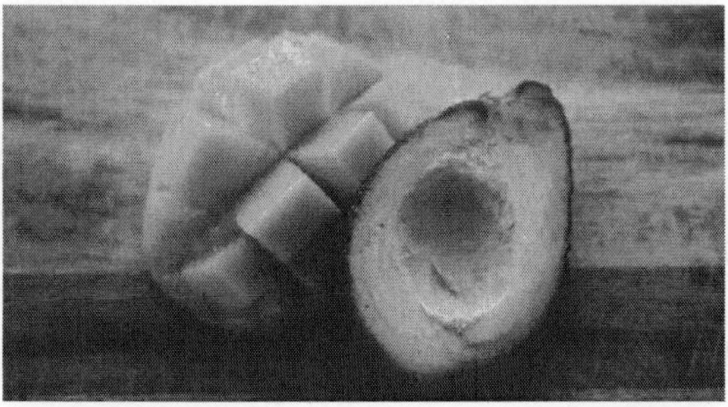

Vitamin A, D, E, and K all are fat-soluble vitamins. These fat-soluble vitamins require the availability of fat to absorb properly in the body. Your body can't absorb them effectively without eating some fat at the same time. Some examples of foods containing fat-soluble vitamins are mango, red bell peppers, sweet potato, and most of the colored vegetables (vitamin A), milk and milk products (Vitamin D), almonds, peanuts, sunflower seeds (vitamin E) and leafy greens like spinach, kale, cauliflower (Vitamin K).

Food combinations that you should eat for better absorption of fat-soluble vitamins:

1. Almond milkshake

2. Nuts roasted in cow's ghee

3. Spinach + Mustard oil

4. Mango + Avocado

5. Nuts + Flaxseeds

CONCLUSION

It is not very hard to eat the food combinations mentioned above. Some of the above food combinations you might already be eating, some combinations might be new to you. It's time to do some experiments with your taste bud. If you come up with a new dish while combining these nutrients, do let me know. I would love to try it too.

5

DIET PLAN FOR HEALTHY AND DISEASE-FREE LIFE

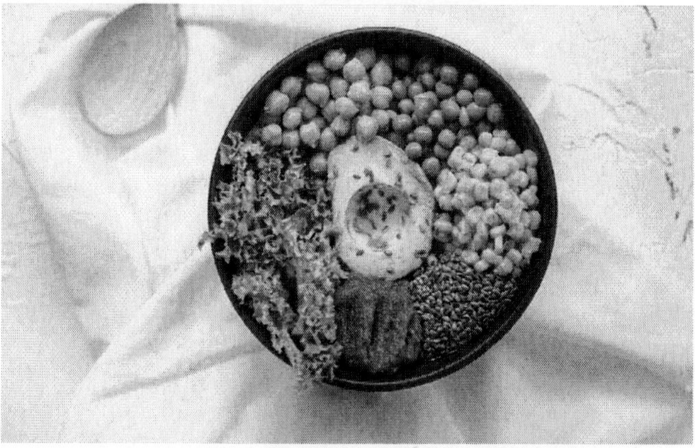

Diet plan for healthy and disease-free life

- Drink lemon water on an empty stomach.
- Eat overnight soaked dry fruits every day.
    - In winter, 8 almonds + 6 cashews + 6 pistachios + 8 raisins + 2 figs + 4 dates.
    - In summer, (Must be soaked overnight) 5-6 almonds + 4 cashews + 4 pistachios + 4 raisins + 1 fig + 2 dates.

- Drink green tea with lemon juice. If you must add sugar, then add jaggery powder instead of sugar in it.
- Add barley flour to your whole wheat flour in a ratio of 1:7. Add 1 kg barley flour in 7 kg of whole wheat flour.
- Drink more water. Water helps remove toxins from your blood through urine.
- Eat one crushed garlic on an empty stomach once in a week.
- Crush fenugreek seeds and use fenugreek powder in cooking. Fenugreek seeds are bitter in taste, so add 1-2 teaspoon only. If you can tolerate the bitter taste, then add up to 1 tablespoon.
- Use spices such as turmeric, cinnamon, and cumin in cooking.
- Eat one flax seeds laddoo (see in the recipes section) every day.
- Use cold-pressed oil in cooking, such as mustard oil instead of refined oil.
- Use three types of oil- mustard oil for cooking, refined oil such as soybean oil for deep frying, and extra virgin olive oil for sautéing or low flame cooking. Don't use olive oil to deep fry.
- Eat a variety of sprouts.

- Eat seasonal fruits and vegetables, eat them in plenty in season avoid eating non-seasonal fruits and vegetables; they are inferior in nutritional content.
- Drink one glass of milk daily no matter what's your age. Milk is not only required for kids, it is a must for all age groups.

NOTE FROM LA FONCEUR

Dear Reader,

Thank you for reading *How to Live Disease-Free with Superfoods*. I hope you have found this book helpful.

If you liked the book, please leave a review online. Help other health-conscious readers find this book by telling them why you enjoyed reading. Your help in spreading awareness will be gratefully received.

Join my mailing list at www.eatsowhat.com/signup

If you are looking for a permanent solution to your hair problems, read *Secret of Healthy Hair*.

Learn how a vegetarian diet can be the solution to a disease-free healthy life in Eat So What! series- *Eat So What! The Power of Vegetarianism* and *Eat So What! Smart Ways to Stay Healthy*.

All of my books are available in eBook, paperback, and hardcover editions.

Regards

La Fonceur

REFERENCES

1. Soheil Z, Habsah A, "A Review on Antibacterial, Antiviral, and Antifungal Activity of Curcumin." Biomed Res Int. 2014; 2014: 186864.
2. Silagy C, Neil A, "Garlic as a lipid lowering agent--a meta-analysis." R Coll Physicians Lond. Jan-Feb 1994;28(1):39-45.
3. Matthias B, Mandy S, "Fiber and magnesium intake and incidence of type 2 diabetes: a prospective study and meta-analysis." Arch Intern Med. 2007 May 14;167(9):956-65.
4. Karin R, Toben C, Fakler P, "Effect of garlic on serum lipids: an updated meta-analysis." Nutr Rev. 2013 May;71(5):282-99.
5. Holly L, Sharon A, "Garlic and onions: Their cancer prevention properties." Cancer Prev Res (Phila). 2015 Mar; 8(3): 181–189.
6. Ranade M, Mudgalkar N, "A simple dietary addition of fenugreek seed leads to the reduction in blood glucose levels: A parallel-group, randomized single-blind trial." Ayu. 2017 Jan-Jun; 38(1-2): 24–27.
7. Calado A, Neves M, "The Effect of Flaxseed in Breast Cancer: A Literature Review." Front Nutr. 2018; 5: 4.

8. Chikako M, Taeko K, "Effects of glycolipids from spinach on mammalian DNA polymerases." Biochem Pharmacol. 2003 Jan 15;65(2):259-67.

9. Mondal S, Varma S, "Double-blinded randomized controlled trial for immunomodulatory effects of Tulsi (Ocimum sanctum Linn.) leaf extract on healthy volunteers." Ethnopharmacol. 2011 Jul 14;136(3):452-

10. Dokania M, Kishore K, Sharma PK, "Effect of Ocimum sanctum extract on sodium nitrite-induced experimental amnesia in mice." Thai J Pharma Sci. 2011; 35:123–30.

11. Eddouks M, Amina B, "Antidiabetic plants improving insulin sensitivity." J Pharm Pharmacol. 2014 Sep;66(9):1197-214.

12. Widjaja S, Rusdiana, "Glucose Lowering Effect of Basil Leaves in Diabetic Rats." J Med Sci. 2019 May 15; 7(9): 1415–1417.

13. A review on, "What You Need to Know about Dietary Supplements." https://www.fda.gov/food/

14. Gallagher J, Vinod Yalamanchili V, "The Effect of Vitamin D on Calcium Absorption in Older Women." J Clin Endocrinol Metab. 2012 Oct; 97(10): 3550–3556.

15. Gupta R, Gangoliya S, "Reduction of phytic acid and enhancement of bioavailable micronutrients in food grains." J Food Sci Technol. 2015 Feb; 52(2): 676–684.

16. Lee A, Thurnham D, "Consumption of tomato products with olive oil but not sunflower oil increases the antioxidant activity of plasma." Free Radical Biol Med. 2000 Nov 15;29(10):1051-5.

17. Malouf M, Grimley E, "Folic acid with or without vitamin B12 for cognition and dementia." Cochrane Database Syst Rev, 2003;(4): CD004514.

18. Abularrage C, Sidawy A, "Effect of folic Acid and vitamins B6 and B12 on microcirculatory vasoreactivity in patients with hyperhomocysteinemia." Vasc Endovascular Surg. 2007 Aug-Sep;41(4):339-45.

19. Sarwar N, Gao P, "Diabetes mellitus, fasting blood glucose concentration, and risk of vascular disease: a collaborative meta-analysis of 102 prospective studies. Emerging Risk Factors Collaboration." Lancet. 2010; 26; 375:2215-2222.

20. Bourne R, Stevens G, "Causes of vision loss worldwide, 1990-2010: a systematic analysis." Lancet Global Health 2013;1:e339-e349

IMPORTANT TERMINOLOGY

Free radicals: Free radicals are the unpaired electrons that form due to the oxidative process in the body. These unpaired electrons like to be in pairs, so they pair with the electrons in proteins and DNA and damage them.

Antioxidants: Body has antioxidants, which neutralize free radicals by inhibiting the oxidative process that forms free radicals.

Oxidative stress: When free radicals outnumber the naturally occurring antioxidants, it results in oxidative stress. This imbalance leads to cell and tissue damage, including DNA, protein, and lipids. Damage to your DNA increases your risk of chronic diseases such as cancer, rheumatoid arthritis, diabetics, stroke, and aging.

Inflammation: Inflammation is the response of the body to harmful pathogens, and irritants, and eliminate the initial cause of cell injury. Body releases white blood cells to heal the damaged cells. When the immune system mistakenly attacks healthy tissue, it causes harmful abnormal inflammation. Reasons for abnormal inflammation are stress, smoking, and alcohol consumption. Some examples of diseases associated with abnormal inflammations are rheumatoid arthritis, psoriasis, and inflammatory bowel diseases.

ABOUT THE AUTHOR

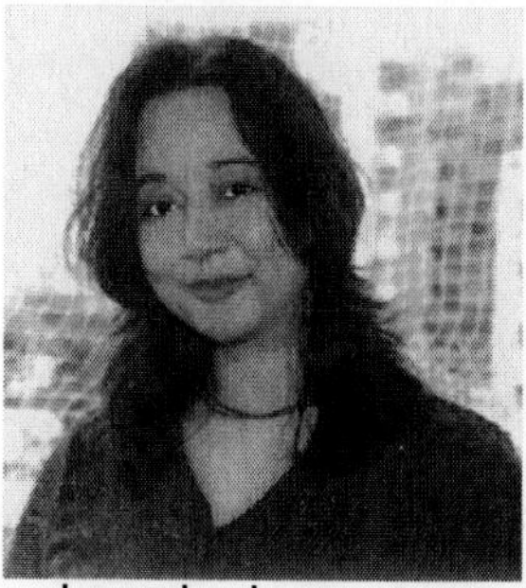

La Fonceur is the author of the book series ***Eat So What!*** and ***Secret of Healthy* Hair**, a dance artist, and a health blogger. She has a master's degree in Pharmacy. She specialized in Pharmaceutical Technology and worked as a research scientist in the research and development department. She has published an article titled 'Techniques for Producing Biotechnology-Derived Products of Pharmaceutical Use' in Pharmtechmedica Journal. She is also a registered pharmacist. Being a research scientist, she has worked closely with drugs. Based on her experience, she believes that one can prevent most of the diseases with nutritious vegetarian foods and a healthy lifestyle.

CONNECT WITH LA FONCEUR

Instagram: **@la_fonceur | @eatsowhat**

Facebook: **LaFonceur | eatsowhatblog**

Twitter: **@la_fonceur**

Sign up to La Fonceur for exclusive offers:

Blog: **www.eatsowhat.com**

Website: **www.lafonceur.com/sign-up**

ALL BOOKS BY LA FONCEUR

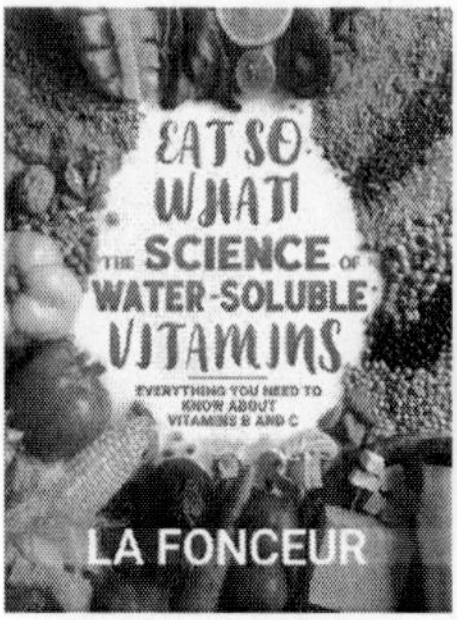

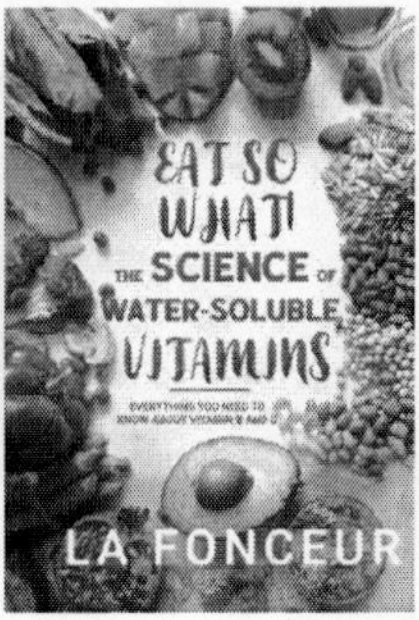

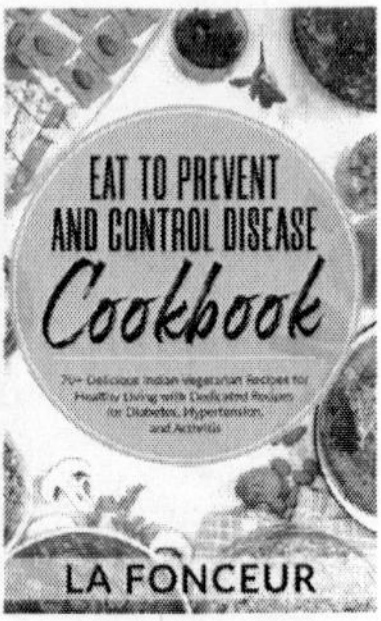

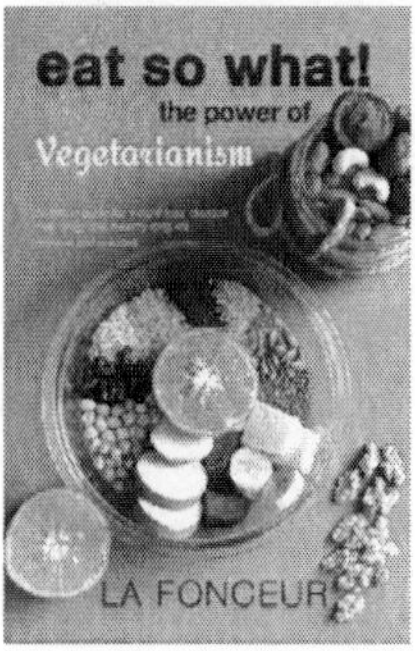

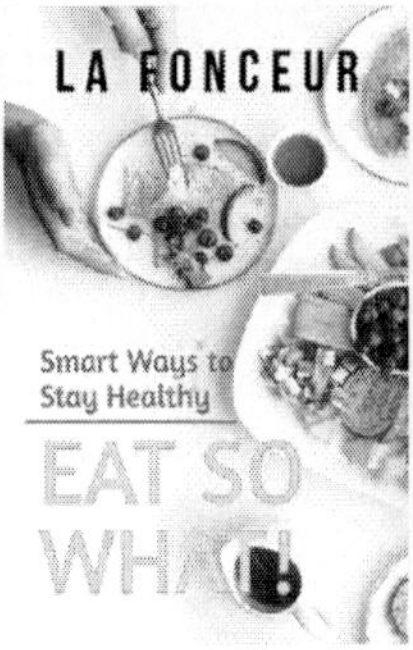

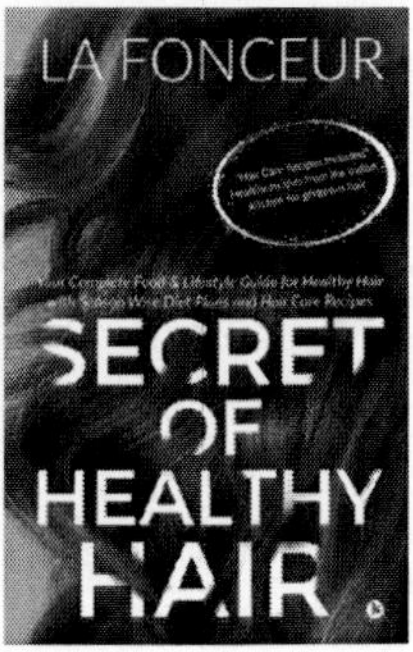

Hindi Editions

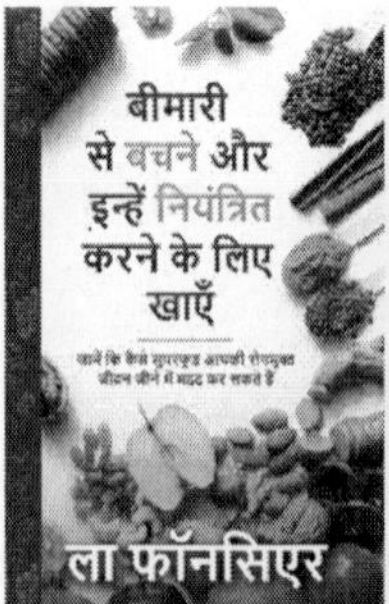

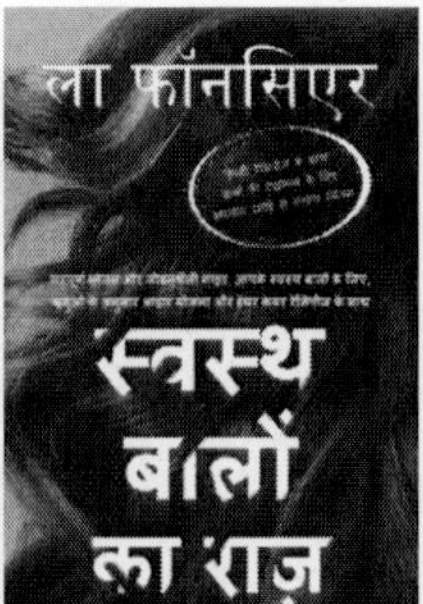

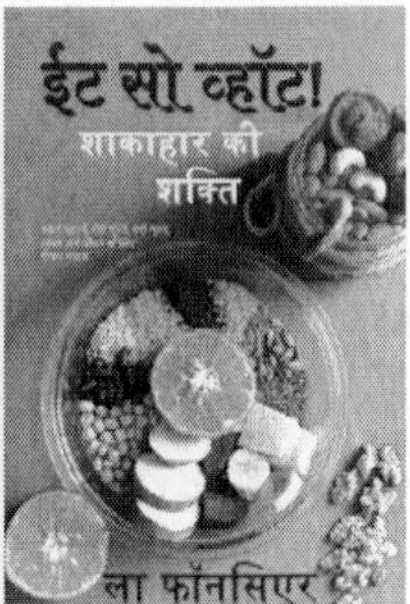